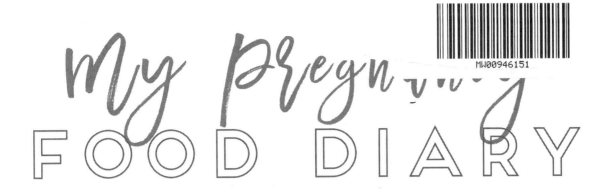

My Pregnancy
FOOD DIARY

Date: _____

Breakfast

Name:

Serving:

Calories:

Carbohydrates:

Protein:

Fat:

Vegetables:

Dairy:

Fiber:

Grains:

How many water intake:

◯ ◯ ◯ ◯ ◯ ◯ ◯ ◯

How hungry were you before eating?

How full were you after eating?

Lunch

Name:

Serving:

Calories:

Carbohydrates:

Protein:

Fat:

Vegetables:

Dairy:

Fiber:

Grains:

How many water intake:

◯ ◯ ◯ ◯ ◯ ◯ ◯ ◯

How hungry were you before eating?

How full were you after eating?

Snacks

Name:
Serving:
Calories:
Carbohydrates:
Protein:
Fat:
Vegetables:
Dairy:
Fiber:

Grains:

How many water intake:

$\bigcirc$ $\bigcirc$ $\bigcirc$ $\bigcirc$ $\bigcirc$ $\bigcirc$ $\bigcirc$ $\bigcirc$

How hungry were you before eating?

How full were you after eating?

Dinner

Name:
Serving:
Calories:
Carbohydrates:
Protein:
Fat:
Vegetables:
Dairy:
Fiber:

Grains:

How many water intake:

◯ ◯ ◯ ◯ ◯ ◯ ◯ ◯

How hungry were you before eating?

How full were you after eating?

Notes

My Pregnancy
FOOD DIARY

Date: _____

Breakfast

Name:

Serving:

Calories:

Carbohydrates:

Protein:

Fat:

Vegetables:

Dairy:

Fiber:

Grains:

How many water intake:

○ ○ ○ ○ ○ ○ ○ ○

How hungry were you before eating?

How full were you after eating?

Lunch

Name:
Serving:
Calories:
Carbohydrates:
Protein:
Fat:
Vegetables:
Dairy:
Fiber:

Grains:

How many water intake:

◯ ◯ ◯ ◯ ◯ ◯ ◯ ◯

How hungry were you before eating?

How full were you after eating?

Snacks

Name:
Serving:
Calories:
Carbohydrates:
Protein:
Fat:
Vegetables:
Dairy:
Fiber:

Grains:

How many water intake:

◯ ◯ ◯ ◯ ◯ ◯ ◯ ◯

How hungry were you before eating?

How full were you after eating?

Dinner

Name:

Serving:

Calories:

Carbohydrates:

Protein:

Fat:

Vegetables:

Dairy:

Fiber:

Grains:

How many water intake:

○ ○ ○ ○ ○ ○ ○ ○

How hungry were you before eating?

How full were you after eating?

Notes

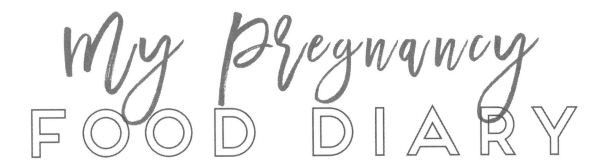

My Pregnancy
FOOD DIARY

Date: _____

Breakfast

Name:

Serving:

Calories:

Carbohydrates:

Protein:

Fat:

Vegetables:

Dairy:

Fiber:

Grains:

How many water intake:

◯ ◯ ◯ ◯ ◯ ◯ ◯ ◯

How hungry were you before eating?

How full were you after eating?

Lunch

Name:

Serving:

Calories:

Carbohydrates:

Protein:

Fat:

Vegetables:

Dairy:

Fiber:

Grains:

How many water intake:

◯ ◯ ◯ ◯ ◯ ◯ ◯ ◯

How hungry were you before eating?

How full were you after eating?

Snacks

Name:
Serving:
Calories:
Carbohydrates:
Protein:
Fat:
Vegetables:
Dairy:
Fiber:

Grains:

How many water intake:

◯ ◯ ◯ ◯ ◯ ◯ ◯ ◯

How hungry were you before eating?

How full were you after eating?

Dinner

Name:
Serving:
Calories:
Carbohydrates:
Protein:
Fat:
Vegetables:
Dairy:
Fiber:

Grains:

How many water intake:

◯ ◯ ◯ ◯ ◯ ◯ ◯ ◯

How hungry were you before eating?

How full were you after eating?

Notes

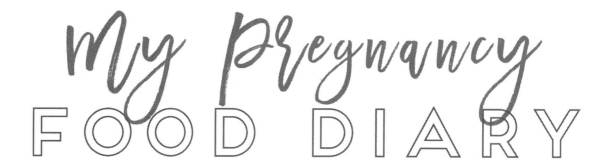

My Pregnancy
FOOD DIARY

Date: _____

Breakfast

Name:

Serving:

Calories:

Carbohydrates:

Protein:

Fat:

Vegetables:

Dairy:

Fiber:

Grains:

How many water intake:

◯ ◯ ◯ ◯ ◯ ◯ ◯ ◯

How hungry were you before eating?

How full were you after eating?

Lunch

Name:

Serving:

Calories:

Carbohydrates:

Protein:

Fat:

Vegetables:

Dairy:

Fiber:

Grains:

How many water intake:

◯ ◯ ◯ ◯ ◯ ◯ ◯ ◯

How hungry were you before eating?

How full were you after eating?

Snacks

Name:
Serving:
Calories:
Carbohydrates:
Protein:
Fat:
Vegetables:
Dairy:
Fiber:

Grains:

How many water intake:

◯ ◯ ◯ ◯ ◯ ◯ ◯ ◯

How hungry were you before eating?

How full were you after eating?

Dinner

Name:

Serving:

Calories:

Carbohydrates:

Protein:

Fat:

Vegetables:

Dairy:

Fiber:

Grains:

How many water intake:

◯ ◯ ◯ ◯ ◯ ◯ ◯ ◯

How hungry were you before eating?

How full were you after eating?

Notes

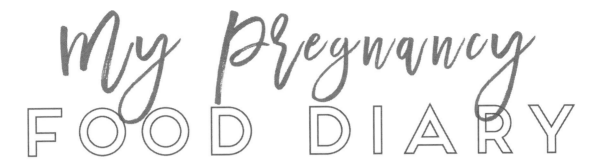

My Pregnancy
FOOD DIARY

Date: _____

Breakfast

Name:

Serving:

Calories:

Carbohydrates:

Protein:

Fat:

Vegetables:

Dairy:

Fiber:

Grains:

How many water intake:

◯ ◯ ◯ ◯ ◯ ◯ ◯ ◯

How hungry were you before eating?

How full were you after eating?

Lunch

Name:
Serving:
Calories:
Carbohydrates:
Protein:
Fat:
Vegetables:
Dairy:
Fiber:

Grains:

How many water intake:

◯ ◯ ◯ ◯ ◯ ◯ ◯ ◯

How hungry were you before eating?

How full were you after eating?

Snacks

Name:

Serving:

Calories:

Carbohydrates:

Protein:

Fat:

Vegetables:

Dairy:

Fiber:

Grains:

How many water intake:

○ ○ ○ ○ ○ ○ ○ ○

How hungry were you before eating?

How full were you after eating?

Dinner

Name:
Serving:
Calories:
Carbohydrates:
Protein:
Fat:
Vegetables:
Dairy:
Fiber:

Grains:

How many water intake:

◯ ◯ ◯ ◯ ◯ ◯ ◯ ◯

How hungry were you before eating?

How full were you after eating?

Notes

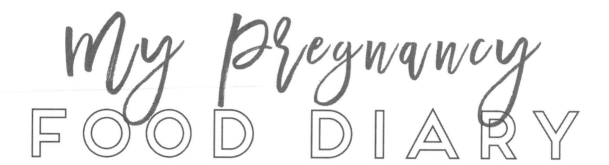

My Pregnancy
FOOD DIARY

Date: _____

Breakfast

Name:

Serving:

Calories:

Carbohydrates:

Protein:

Fat:

Vegetables:

Dairy:

Fiber:

Grains:

How many water intake:

◯ ◯ ◯ ◯ ◯ ◯ ◯ ◯

How hungry were you before eating?

How full were you after eating?

Lunch

Name:
Serving:
Calories:
Carbohydrates:
Protein:
Fat:
Vegetables:
Dairy:
Fiber:

Grains:

How many water intake:

◯ ◯ ◯ ◯ ◯ ◯ ◯ ◯

How hungry were you before eating?

How full were you after eating?

Snacks

Name:
Serving:
Calories:
Carbohydrates:
Protein:
Fat:
Vegetables:
Dairy:
Fiber:

Grains:

How many water intake:

◯ ◯ ◯ ◯ ◯ ◯ ◯ ◯

How hungry were you before eating?

How full were you after eating?

Dinner

Name:
Serving:
Calories:
Carbohydrates:
Protein:
Fat:
Vegetables:
Dairy:
Fiber:

Grains:

How many water intake:

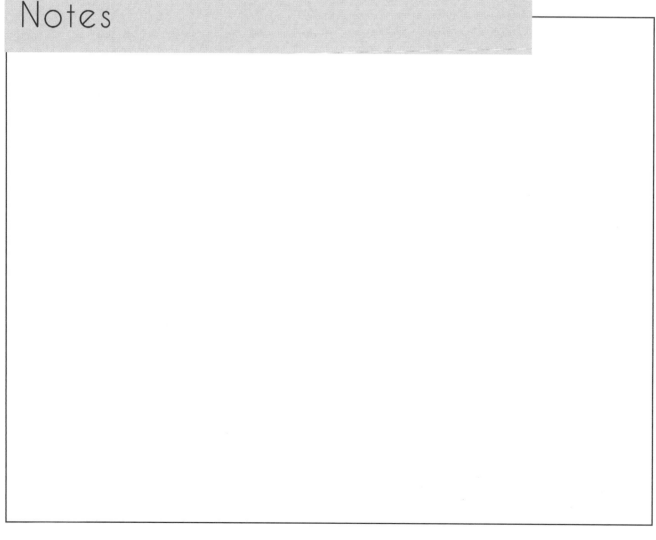

How hungry were you before eating?

How full were you after eating?

Notes

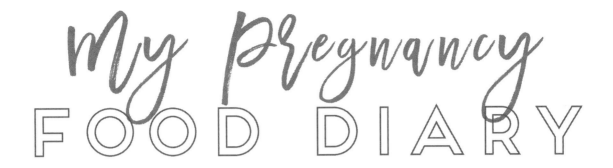

My Pregnancy
FOOD DIARY

Date: _____

Breakfast

Name:

Serving:

Calories:

Carbohydrates:

Protein:

Fat:

Vegetables:

Dairy:

Fiber:

Grains:

How many water intake:

◯ ◯ ◯ ◯ ◯ ◯ ◯ ◯

How hungry were you before eating?

How full were you after eating?

Lunch

Name:
Serving:
Calories:
Carbohydrates:
Protein:
Fat:
Vegetables:
Dairy:
Fiber:

Grains:

How many water intake:

◯ ◯ ◯ ◯ ◯ ◯ ◯ ◯

How hungry were you before eating?

How full were you after eating?

Snacks

Name:
Serving:
Calories:
Carbohydrates:
Protein:
Fat:
Vegetables:
Dairy:
Fiber:

Grains:

How many water intake:

◯ ◯ ◯ ◯ ◯ ◯ ◯ ◯

How hungry were you before eating?

How full were you after eating?

Dinner

Name:
Serving:
Calories:
Carbohydrates:
Protein:
Fat:
Vegetables:
Dairy:
Fiber:

Grains:

How many water intake:

◯ ◯ ◯ ◯ ◯ ◯ ◯ ◯

How hungry were you before eating?

How full were you after eating?

Notes

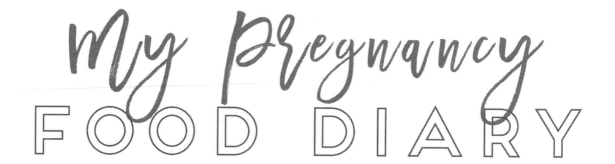

My Pregnancy
FOOD DIARY

Date: _____

Breakfast

Name:

Serving:

Calories:

Carbohydrates:

Protein:

Fat:

Vegetables:

Dairy:

Fiber:

Grains:

How many water intake:

◯ ◯ ◯ ◯ ◯ ◯ ◯ ◯

How hungry were you before eating?

How full were you after eating?

Lunch

Name:

Serving:

Calories:

Carbohydrates:

Protein:

Fat:

Vegetables:

Dairy:

Fiber:

Grains:

How many water intake:

○ ○ ○ ○ ○ ○ ○ ○

How hungry were you before eating?

How full were you after eating?

Snacks

Name:
Serving:
Calories:
Carbohydrates:
Protein:
Fat:
Vegetables:
Dairy:
Fiber:

Grains:

How many water intake:

◯ ◯ ◯ ◯ ◯ ◯ ◯ ◯

How hungry were you before eating?

How full were you after eating?

Dinner

Name:
Serving:
Calories:
Carbohydrates:
Protein:
Fat:
Vegetables:
Dairy:
Fiber:

Grains:

How many water intake:

◯ ◯ ◯ ◯ ◯ ◯ ◯ ◯

How hungry were you before eating?

How full were you after eating?

Notes

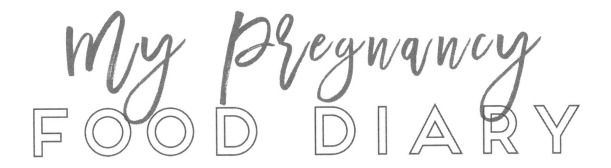

My Pregnancy
FOOD DIARY

Date: _____

Breakfast

Name:

Serving:

Calories:

Carbohydrates:

Protein:

Fat:

Vegetables:

Dairy:

Fiber:

Grains:

How many water intake:

◯ ◯ ◯ ◯ ◯ ◯ ◯ ◯

How hungry were you before eating?

How full were you after eating?

Lunch

Name:

Serving:

Calories:

Carbohydrates:

Protein:

Fat:

Vegetables:

Dairy:

Fiber:

Grains:

How many water intake:

◯ ◯ ◯ ◯ ◯ ◯ ◯ ◯

How hungry were you before eating?

How full were you after eating?

Snacks

Name:
Serving:
Calories:
Carbohydrates:
Protein:
Fat:
Vegetables:
Dairy:
Fiber:

Grains:

How many water intake:

◯ ◯ ◯ ◯ ◯ ◯ ◯ ◯

How hungry were you before eating?

How full were you after eating?

Dinner

Name:
Serving:
Calories:
Carbohydrates:
Protein:
Fat:
Vegetables:
Dairy:
Fiber:

Grains:

How many water intake:

◯ ◯ ◯ ◯ ◯ ◯ ◯ ◯

How hungry were you before eating?

How full were you after eating?

Notes

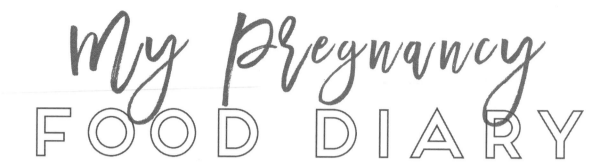

My Pregnancy
FOOD DIARY

Date: _____

Breakfast

Name:

Serving:

Calories:

Carbohydrates:

Protein:

Fat:

Vegetables:

Dairy:

Fiber:

Grains:

How many water intake:

○ ○ ○ ○ ○ ○ ○ ○

How hungry were you before eating?

How full were you after eating?

Lunch

Name:
Serving:
Calories:
Carbohydrates:
Protein:
Fat:
Vegetables:
Dairy:
Fiber:

Grains:

How many water intake:

◯ ◯ ◯ ◯ ◯ ◯ ◯ ◯

How hungry were you before eating?

How full were you after eating?

Snacks

Name:
Serving:
Calories:
Carbohydrates:
Protein:
Fat:
Vegetables:
Dairy:
Fiber:

Grains:

How many water intake:

◯ ◯ ◯ ◯ ◯ ◯ ◯ ◯

How hungry were you before eating?

How full were you after eating?

Dinner

Name:
Serving:
Calories:
Carbohydrates:
Protein:
Fat:
Vegetables:
Dairy:
Fiber:

Grains:

How many water intake:

◯ ◯ ◯ ◯ ◯ ◯ ◯ ◯

How hungry were you before eating?

How full were you after eating?

Notes

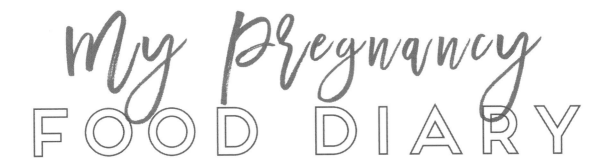
My Pregnancy
FOOD DIARY

Date: _____

Breakfast

Name:
Serving:
Calories:
Carbohydrates:
Protein:
Fat:
Vegetables:
Dairy:
Fiber:
Grains:

How many water intake:

○　○　○　○　○　○　○　○

How hungry were you before eating?

How full were you after eating?

Lunch

Name:

Serving:

Calories:

Carbohydrates:

Protein:

Fat:

Vegetables:

Dairy:

Fiber:

Grains:

How many water intake:

◯ ◯ ◯ ◯ ◯ ◯ ◯ ◯

How hungry were you before eating?

How full were you after eating?

Snacks

Name:
Serving:
Calories:
Carbohydrates:
Protein:
Fat:
Vegetables:
Dairy:
Fiber:

Grains:

How many water intake:

○ ○ ○ ○ ○ ○ ○ ○

How hungry were you before eating?

How full were you after eating?

Dinner

Name:
Serving:
Calories:
Carbohydrates:
Protein:
Fat:
Vegetables:
Dairy:
Fiber:

Grains:

How many water intake:

○ ○ ○ ○ ○ ○ ○ ○

How hungry were you before eating?

How full were you after eating?

Notes

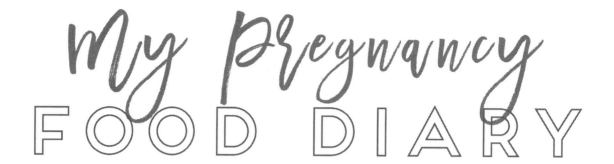

My Pregnancy
FOOD DIARY

Date: _____

Breakfast

Name:

Serving:

Calories:

Carbohydrates:

Protein:

Fat:

Vegetables:

Dairy:

Fiber:

Grains:

How many water intake:

○ ○ ○ ○ ○ ○ ○ ○

How hungry were you before eating?

How full were you after eating?

Lunch

Name:
Serving:
Calories:
Carbohydrates:
Protein:
Fat:
Vegetables:
Dairy:
Fiber:

Grains:

How many water intake:

◯ ◯ ◯ ◯ ◯ ◯ ◯ ◯

How hungry were you before eating?

How full were you after eating?

Snacks

Name:
Serving:
Calories:
Carbohydrates:
Protein:
Fat:
Vegetables:
Dairy:
Fiber:

Grains:

How many water intake:

◯ ◯ ◯ ◯ ◯ ◯ ◯ ◯

How hungry were you before eating?

How full were you after eating?

Dinner

Name:
Serving:
Calories:
Carbohydrates:
Protein:
Fat:
Vegetables:
Dairy:
Fiber:

Grains:

How many water intake:

◯ ◯ ◯ ◯ ◯ ◯ ◯ ◯

How hungry were you before eating?

How full were you after eating?

Notes

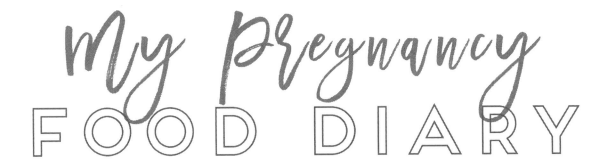

My Pregnancy
FOOD DIARY

Date: _____

Breakfast

Name:

Serving:

Calories:

Carbohydrates:

Protein:

Fat:

Vegetables:

Dairy:

Fiber:

Grains:

How many water intake:

○ ○ ○ ○ ○ ○ ○ ○

How hungry were you before eating?

How full were you after eating?

Lunch

Name:

Serving:

Calories:

Carbohydrates:

Protein:

Fat:

Vegetables:

Dairy:

Fiber:

Grains:

How many water intake:

◯ ◯ ◯ ◯ ◯ ◯ ◯ ◯

How hungry were you before eating?

How full were you after eating?

Snacks

Name:
Serving:
Calories:
Carbohydrates:
Protein:
Fat:
Vegetables:
Dairy:
Fiber:

Grains:

How many water intake:

◯ ◯ ◯ ◯ ◯ ◯ ◯ ◯

How hungry were you before eating?

How full were you after eating?

Dinner

Name:
Serving:
Calories:
Carbohydrates:
Protein:
Fat:
Vegetables:
Dairy:
Fiber:

Grains:

How many water intake:

◯ ◯ ◯ ◯ ◯ ◯ ◯ ◯

How hungry were you before eating?

How full were you after eating?

Notes

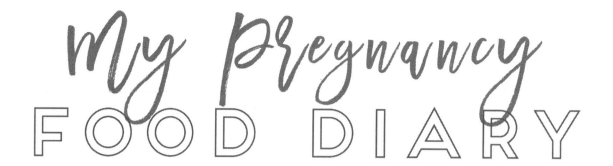

My Pregnancy
FOOD DIARY

Date: _____

Breakfast

Name:

Serving:

Calories:

Carbohydrates:

Protein:

Fat:

Vegetables:

Dairy:

Fiber:

Grains:

How many water intake:

◯ ◯ ◯ ◯ ◯ ◯ ◯ ◯

How hungry were you before eating?

How full were you after eating?

Lunch

Name:
Serving:
Calories:
Carbohydrates:
Protein:
Fat:
Vegetables:
Dairy:
Fiber:

Grains:

How many water intake:

◯ ◯ ◯ ◯ ◯ ◯ ◯ ◯

How hungry were you before eating?

How full were you after eating?

Snacks

Name:
Serving:
Calories:
Carbohydrates:
Protein:
Fat:
Vegetables:
Dairy:
Fiber:

Grains:

How many water intake:

◯ ◯ ◯ ◯ ◯ ◯ ◯ ◯

How hungry were you before eating?

How full were you after eating?

Dinner

Name:
Serving:
Calories:
Carbohydrates:
Protein:
Fat:
Vegetables:
Dairy:
Fiber:

Grains:

How many water intake:

◯ ◯ ◯ ◯ ◯ ◯ ◯ ◯

How hungry were you before eating?

How full were you after eating?

Notes

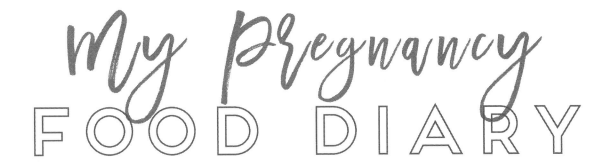

My Pregnancy
FOOD DIARY

Date: _____

Breakfast

Name:

Serving:

Calories:

Carbohydrates:

Protein:

Fat:

Vegetables:

Dairy:

Fiber:

Grains:

How many water intake:

◯ ◯ ◯ ◯ ◯ ◯ ◯ ◯

How hungry were you before eating?

How full were you after eating?

Lunch

Name:
Serving:
Calories:
Carbohydrates:
Protein:
Fat:
Vegetables:
Dairy:
Fiber:

Grains:

How many water intake:

◯ ◯ ◯ ◯ ◯ ◯ ◯ ◯

How hungry were you before eating?

How full were you after eating?

Snacks

Name:
Serving:
Calories:
Carbohydrates:
Protein:
Fat:
Vegetables:
Dairy:
Fiber:

Grains:

How many water intake:

◯ ◯ ◯ ◯ ◯ ◯ ◯ ◯

How hungry were you before eating?

How full were you after eating?

Dinner

Name:
Serving:
Calories:
Carbohydrates:
Protein:
Fat:
Vegetables:
Dairy:
Fiber:

Grains:

How many water intake:

○ ○ ○ ○ ○ ○ ○ ○

How hungry were you before eating?

How full were you after eating?

Notes

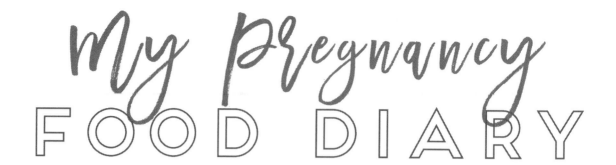

My Pregnancy
FOOD DIARY

Date: _____

Breakfast

Name:

Serving:

Calories:

Carbohydrates:

Protein:

Fat:

Vegetables:

Dairy:

Fiber:

Grains:

How many water intake:

◯ ◯ ◯ ◯ ◯ ◯ ◯ ◯

How hungry were you before eating?

How full were you after eating?

Lunch

Name:

Serving:

Calories:

Carbohydrates:

Protein:

Fat:

Vegetables:

Dairy:

Fiber:

Grains:

How many water intake:

◯ ◯ ◯ ◯ ◯ ◯ ◯ ◯

How hungry were you before eating?

How full were you after eating?

Snacks

Name:
Serving:
Calories:
Carbohydrates:
Protein:
Fat:
Vegetables:
Dairy:
Fiber:

Grains:

How many water intake:

◯ ◯ ◯ ◯ ◯ ◯ ◯ ◯

How hungry were you before eating?

How full were you after eating?

Dinner

Name:

Serving:

Calories:

Carbohydrates:

Protein:

Fat:

Vegetables:

Dairy:

Fiber:

Grains:

How many water intake:

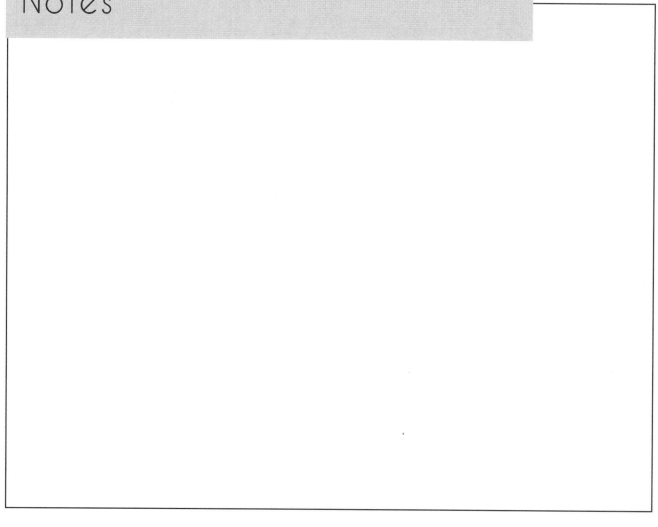

How hungry were you before eating?

How full were you after eating?

Notes

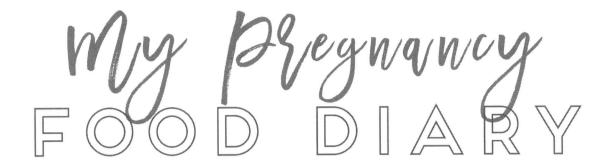

My Pregnancy
FOOD DIARY

Date: _____

Breakfast

Name:
Serving:
Calories:
Carbohydrates:
Protein:
Fat:
Vegetables:
Dairy:
Fiber:
Grains:

How many water intake:

◯ ◯ ◯ ◯ ◯ ◯ ◯ ◯

How hungry were you before eating?

How full were you after eating?

Lunch

Name:

Serving:

Calories:

Carbohydrates:

Protein:

Fat:

Vegetables:

Dairy:

Fiber:

Grains:

How many water intake:

◯ ◯ ◯ ◯ ◯ ◯ ◯ ◯

How hungry were you before eating?

How full were you after eating?

Snacks

Name:

Serving:

Calories:

Carbohydrates:

Protein:

Fat:

Vegetables:

Dairy:

Fiber:

Grains:

How many water intake:

◯ ◯ ◯ ◯ ◯ ◯ ◯ ◯

How hungry were you before eating?

How full were you after eating?

Dinner

Name:
Serving:
Calories:
Carbohydrates:
Protein:
Fat:
Vegetables:
Dairy:
Fiber:

Grains:

How many water intake:

○ ○ ○ ○ ○ ○ ○ ○

How hungry were you before eating?

How full were you after eating?

Notes

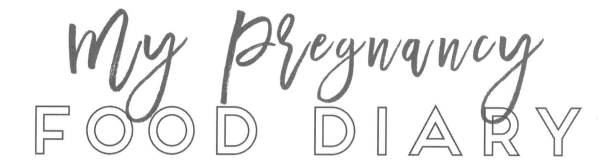

My Pregnancy
FOOD DIARY

Date: _____

Breakfast

Name:

Serving:

Calories:

Carbohydrates:

Protein:

Fat:

Vegetables:

Dairy:

Fiber:

Grains:

How many water intake:

○ ○ ○ ○ ○ ○ ○ ○

How hungry were you before eating?

How full were you after eating?

Lunch

Name:
Serving:
Calories:
Carbohydrates:
Protein:
Fat:
Vegetables:
Dairy:
Fiber:

Grains:

How many water intake:

○ ○ ○ ○ ○ ○ ○ ○

How hungry were you before eating?

How full were you after eating?

Snacks

Name:
Serving:
Calories:
Carbohydrates:
Protein:
Fat:
Vegetables:
Dairy:
Fiber:

Grains:

How many water intake:

◯ ◯ ◯ ◯ ◯ ◯ ◯ ◯

How hungry were you before eating?

How full were you after eating?

Dinner

Name:
Serving:
Calories:
Carbohydrates:
Protein:
Fat:
Vegetables:
Dairy:
Fiber:

Grains:

How many water intake:

◯ ◯ ◯ ◯ ◯ ◯ ◯ ◯

How hungry were you before eating?

How full were you after eating?

Notes

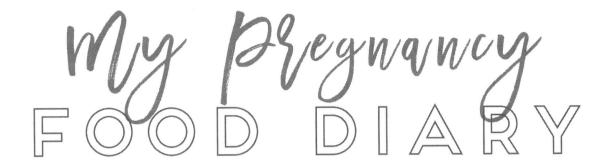

My Pregnancy
FOOD DIARY

Date: _____

Breakfast

Name:

Serving:

Calories:

Carbohydrates:

Protein:

Fat:

Vegetables:

Dairy:

Fiber:

Grains:

How many water intake:

◯ ◯ ◯ ◯ ◯ ◯ ◯ ◯

How hungry were you before eating?

How full were you after eating?

Lunch

Name:

Serving:

Calories:

Carbohydrates:

Protein:

Fat:

Vegetables:

Dairy:

Fiber:

Grains:

How many water intake:

◯ ◯ ◯ ◯ ◯ ◯ ◯ ◯

How hungry were you before eating?

How full were you after eating?

Snacks

Name:
Serving:
Calories:
Carbohydrates:
Protein:
Fat:
Vegetables:
Dairy:
Fiber:

Grains:

How many water intake:

○ ○ ○ ○ ○ ○ ○ ○

How hungry were you before eating?

How full were you after eating?

Dinner

Name:
Serving:
Calories:
Carbohydrates:
Protein:
Fat:
Vegetables:
Dairy:
Fiber:

Grains:

How many water intake:

○ ○ ○ ○ ○ ○ ○ ○

How hungry were you before eating?

How full were you after eating?

Notes

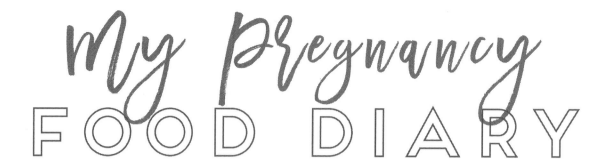

My Pregnancy
FOOD DIARY

Date: _____

Breakfast

Name:

Serving:

Calories:

Carbohydrates:

Protein:

Fat:

Vegetables:

Dairy:

Fiber:

Grains:

How many water intake:

◯ ◯ ◯ ◯ ◯ ◯ ◯ ◯

How hungry were you before eating?

How full were you after eating?

Lunch

Name:
Serving:
Calories:
Carbohydrates:
Protein:
Fat:
Vegetables:
Dairy:
Fiber:

Grains:

How many water intake:

○ ○ ○ ○ ○ ○ ○ ○

How hungry were you before eating?

How full were you after eating?

Snacks

Name:
Serving:
Calories:
Carbohydrates:
Protein:
Fat:
Vegetables:
Dairy:
Fiber:

Grains:

How many water intake:

○ ○ ○ ○ ○ ○ ○ ○

How hungry were you before eating?

How full were you after eating?

Dinner

Name:
Serving:
Calories:
Carbohydrates:
Protein:
Fat:
Vegetables:
Dairy:
Fiber:

Grains:

How many water intake:

◯ ◯ ◯ ◯ ◯ ◯ ◯ ◯

How hungry were you before eating?

How full were you after eating?

Notes

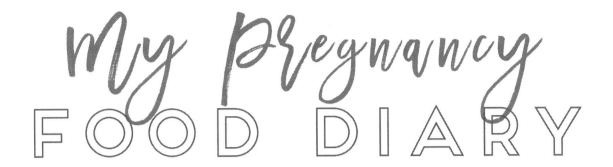

My Pregnancy
FOOD DIARY

Date: _____

Breakfast

Name:

Serving:

Calories:

Carbohydrates:

Protein:

Fat:

Vegetables:

Dairy:

Fiber:

Grains:

How many water intake:

◯ ◯ ◯ ◯ ◯ ◯ ◯ ◯

How hungry were you before eating?

How full were you after eating?

Lunch

Name:
Serving:
Calories:
Carbohydrates:
Protein:
Fat:
Vegetables:
Dairy:
Fiber:

Grains:

How many water intake:

○ ○ ○ ○ ○ ○ ○ ○

How hungry were you before eating?

How full were you after eating?

Snacks

Name:
Serving:
Calories:
Carbohydrates:
Protein:
Fat:
Vegetables:
Dairy:
Fiber:

Grains:

How many water intake:

◯ ◯ ◯ ◯ ◯ ◯ ◯ ◯

How hungry were you before eating?

How full were you after eating?

Dinner

Name:
Serving:
Calories:
Carbohydrates:
Protein:
Fat:
Vegetables:
Dairy:
Fiber:

Grains:

How many water intake:

○ ○ ○ ○ ○ ○ ○ ○

How hungry were you before eating?

How full were you after eating?

Notes

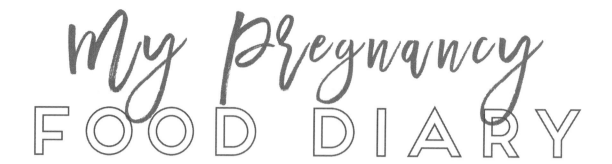

My Pregnancy
FOOD DIARY

Date: _____

Breakfast

Name:

Serving:

Calories:

Carbohydrates:

Protein:

Fat:

Vegetables:

Dairy:

Fiber:

Grains:

How many water intake:

◯ ◯ ◯ ◯ ◯ ◯ ◯ ◯

How hungry were you before eating?

How full were you after eating?

Lunch

Name:
Serving:
Calories:
Carbohydrates:
Protein:
Fat:
Vegetables:
Dairy:
Fiber:

Grains:

How many water intake:

◯ ◯ ◯ ◯ ◯ ◯ ◯ ◯

How hungry were you before eating?

How full were you after eating?

Snacks

Name:
Serving:
Calories:
Carbohydrates:
Protein:
Fat:
Vegetables:
Dairy:
Fiber:

Grains:

How many water intake:

○ ○ ○ ○ ○ ○ ○ ○

How hungry were you before eating?

How full were you after eating?

Dinner

Name:
Serving:
Calories:
Carbohydrates:
Protein:
Fat:
Vegetables:
Dairy:
Fiber:

Grains:

How many water intake:

How hungry were you before eating?

How full were you after eating?

Notes

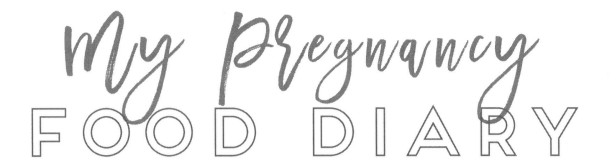

My Pregnancy
FOOD DIARY

Date: _____

Breakfast

Name:

Serving:

Calories:

Carbohydrates:

Protein:

Fat:

Vegetables:

Dairy:

Fiber:

Grains:

How many water intake:

○ ○ ○ ○ ○ ○ ○ ○

How hungry were you before eating?

How full were you after eating?

Lunch

Name:
Serving:
Calories:
Carbohydrates:
Protein:
Fat:
Vegetables:
Dairy:
Fiber:

Grains:

How many water intake:

◯ ◯ ◯ ◯ ◯ ◯ ◯ ◯

How hungry were you before eating?

How full were you after eating?

Snacks

Name:
Serving:
Calories:
Carbohydrates:
Protein:
Fat:
Vegetables:
Dairy:
Fiber:

Grains:

How many water intake:

◯ ◯ ◯ ◯ ◯ ◯ ◯ ◯

How hungry were you before eating?

How full were you after eating?

Dinner

Name:
Serving:
Calories:
Carbohydrates:
Protein:
Fat:
Vegetables:
Dairy:
Fiber:

Grains:

How many water intake:

○ ○ ○ ○ ○ ○ ○ ○

How hungry were you before eating?

How full were you after eating?

Notes

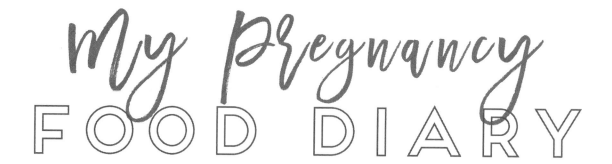

My Pregnancy
FOOD DIARY

Date: _____

Breakfast

Name:

Serving:

Calories:

Carbohydrates:

Protein:

Fat:

Vegetables:

Dairy:

Fiber:

Grains:

How many water intake:

◯ ◯ ◯ ◯ ◯ ◯ ◯ ◯

How hungry were you before eating?

How full were you after eating?

Lunch

Name:

Serving:

Calories:

Carbohydrates:

Protein:

Fat:

Vegetables:

Dairy:

Fiber:

Grains:

How many water intake:

◯ ◯ ◯ ◯ ◯ ◯ ◯ ◯

How hungry were you before eating?

How full were you after eating?

Snacks

Name:
Serving:
Calories:
Carbohydrates:
Protein:
Fat:
Vegetables:
Dairy:
Fiber:

Grains:

How many water intake:

◯ ◯ ◯ ◯ ◯ ◯ ◯ ◯

How hungry were you before eating?

How full were you after eating?

Dinner

Name:

Serving:

Calories:

Carbohydrates:

Protein:

Fat:

Vegetables:

Dairy:

Fiber:

Grains:

How many water intake:

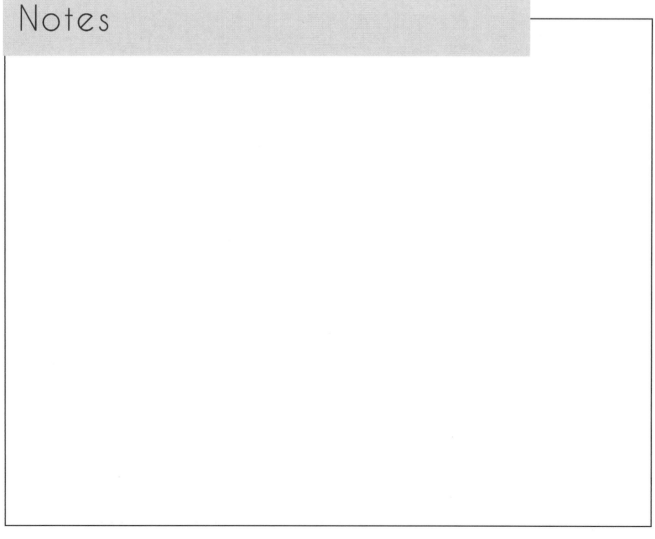

How hungry were you before eating?

How full were you after eating?

Notes

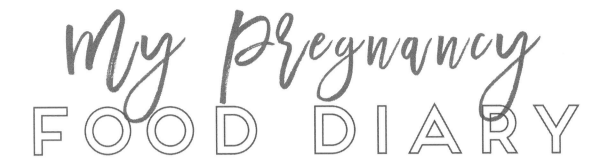

My Pregnancy
FOOD DIARY

Date: _____

Breakfast

Name:

Serving:

Calories:

Carbohydrates:

Protein:

Fat:

Vegetables:

Dairy:

Fiber:

Grains:

How many water intake:

◯ ◯ ◯ ◯ ◯ ◯ ◯ ◯

How hungry were you before eating?

How full were you after eating?

Lunch

Name:
Serving:
Calories:
Carbohydrates:
Protein:
Fat:
Vegetables:
Dairy:
Fiber:

Grains:

How many water intake:

○ ○ ○ ○ ○ ○ ○ ○

How hungry were you before eating?

How full were you after eating?

Snacks

Name:
Serving:
Calories:
Carbohydrates:
Protein:
Fat:
Vegetables:
Dairy:
Fiber:

Grains:

How many water intake:

◯ ◯ ◯ ◯ ◯ ◯ ◯ ◯

How hungry were you before eating?

How full were you after eating?

Dinner

Name:
Serving:
Calories:
Carbohydrates:
Protein:
Fat:
Vegetables:
Dairy:
Fiber:

Grains:

How many water intake:

How hungry were you before eating?

How full were you after eating?

Notes

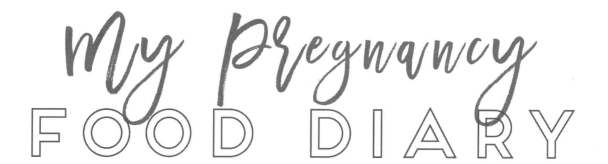

My Pregnancy
FOOD DIARY

Date: _____

Breakfast

Name:

Serving:

Calories:

Carbohydrates:

Protein:

Fat:

Vegetables:

Dairy:

Fiber:

Grains:

How many water intake:

◯ ◯ ◯ ◯ ◯ ◯ ◯ ◯

How hungry were you before eating?

How full were you after eating?

Lunch

Name:

Serving:

Calories:

Carbohydrates:

Protein:

Fat:

Vegetables:

Dairy:

Fiber:

Grains:

How many water intake:

○　○　○　○　○　○　○　○

How hungry were you before eating?

How full were you after eating?

Snacks

Name:

Serving:

Calories:

Carbohydrates:

Protein:

Fat:

Vegetables:

Dairy:

Fiber:

Grains:

How many water intake:

$\bigcirc$ $\bigcirc$ $\bigcirc$ $\bigcirc$ $\bigcirc$ $\bigcirc$ $\bigcirc$ $\bigcirc$

How hungry were you before eating?

How full were you after eating?

Dinner

Name:
Serving:
Calories:
Carbohydrates:
Protein:
Fat:
Vegetables:
Dairy:
Fiber:

Grains:

How many water intake:

○ ○ ○ ○ ○ ○ ○ ○

How hungry were you before eating?

How full were you after eating?

Notes

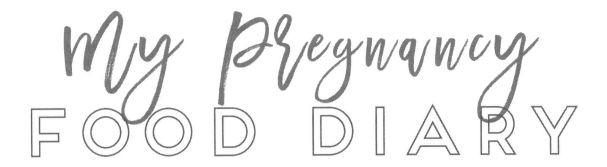

My Pregnancy
FOOD DIARY

Date: _____

Breakfast

Name:

Serving:

Calories:

Carbohydrates:

Protein:

Fat:

Vegetables:

Dairy:

Fiber:

Grains:

How many water intake:

◯ ◯ ◯ ◯ ◯ ◯ ◯ ◯

How hungry were you before eating?

How full were you after eating?

Lunch

Name:

Serving:

Calories:

Carbohydrates:

Protein:

Fat:

Vegetables:

Dairy:

Fiber:

Grains:

How many water intake:

◯ ◯ ◯ ◯ ◯ ◯ ◯ ◯

How hungry were you before eating?

How full were you after eating?

Snacks

Name:
Serving:
Calories:
Carbohydrates:
Protein:
Fat:
Vegetables:
Dairy:
Fiber:

Grains:

How many water intake:

◯ ◯ ◯ ◯ ◯ ◯ ◯ ◯

How hungry were you before eating?

How full were you after eating?

Dinner

Name:
Serving:
Calories:
Carbohydrates:
Protein:
Fat:
Vegetables:
Dairy:
Fiber:

Grains:

How many water intake:

◯ ◯ ◯ ◯ ◯ ◯ ◯ ◯

How hungry were you before eating?

How full were you after eating?

Notes

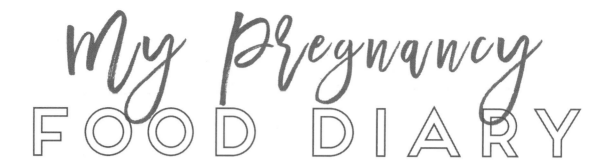

My Pregnancy
FOOD DIARY

Date: _____

Breakfast

Name:

Serving:

Calories:

Carbohydrates:

Protein:

Fat:

Vegetables:

Dairy:

Fiber:

Grains:

How many water intake:

◯ ◯ ◯ ◯ ◯ ◯ ◯ ◯

How hungry were you before eating?

How full were you after eating?

Lunch

Name:

Serving:

Calories:

Carbohydrates:

Protein:

Fat:

Vegetables:

Dairy:

Fiber:

Grains:

How many water intake:

◯ ◯ ◯ ◯ ◯ ◯ ◯ ◯

How hungry were you before eating?

How full were you after eating?

Snacks

Name:
Serving:
Calories:
Carbohydrates:
Protein:
Fat:
Vegetables:
Dairy:
Fiber:

Grains:

How many water intake:

○ ○ ○ ○ ○ ○ ○ ○

How hungry were you before eating?

How full were you after eating?

Dinner

Name:
Serving:
Calories:
Carbohydrates:
Protein:
Fat:
Vegetables:
Dairy:
Fiber:

Grains:

How many water intake:

◯ ◯ ◯ ◯ ◯ ◯ ◯ ◯

How hungry were you before eating?

How full were you after eating?

Notes

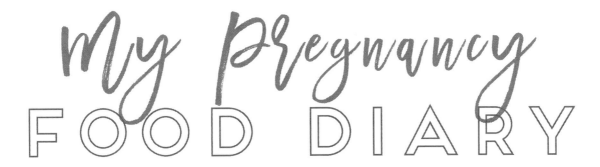

My Pregnancy
FOOD DIARY

Date: _____

Breakfast

Name:

Serving:

Calories:

Carbohydrates:

Protein:

Fat:

Vegetables:

Dairy:

Fiber:

Grains:

How many water intake:

◯ ◯ ◯ ◯ ◯ ◯ ◯ ◯

How hungry were you before eating?

How full were you after eating?

Lunch

Name:

Serving:

Calories:

Carbohydrates:

Protein:

Fat:

Vegetables:

Dairy:

Fiber:

Grains:

How many water intake:

◯ ◯ ◯ ◯ ◯ ◯ ◯ ◯

How hungry were you before eating?

How full were you after eating?

Snacks

Name:
Serving:
Calories:
Carbohydrates:
Protein:
Fat:
Vegetables:
Dairy:
Fiber:

Grains:

How many water intake:

◯ ◯ ◯ ◯ ◯ ◯ ◯ ◯

How hungry were you before eating?

How full were you after eating?

Dinner

Name:
Serving:
Calories:
Carbohydrates:
Protein:
Fat:
Vegetables:
Dairy:
Fiber:

Grains:

How many water intake:

How hungry were you before eating?

How full were you after eating?

Notes

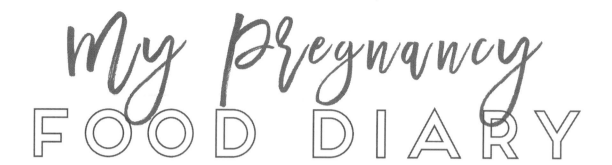

My Pregnancy
FOOD DIARY

Date: _____

Breakfast

Name:

Serving:

Calories:

Carbohydrates:

Protein:

Fat:

Vegetables:

Dairy:

Fiber:

Grains:

How many water intake:

○ ○ ○ ○ ○ ○ ○ ○

How hungry were you before eating?

How full were you after eating?

Lunch

Name:
Serving:
Calories:
Carbohydrates:
Protein:
Fat:
Vegetables:
Dairy:
Fiber:

Grains:

How many water intake:

◯ ◯ ◯ ◯ ◯ ◯ ◯ ◯

How hungry were you before eating?

How full were you after eating?

Snacks

Name:
Serving:
Calories:
Carbohydrates:
Protein:
Fat:
Vegetables:
Dairy:
Fiber:

Grains:

How many water intake:

○ ○ ○ ○ ○ ○ ○ ○

How hungry were you before eating?

How full were you after eating?

Dinner

Name:
Serving:
Calories:
Carbohydrates:
Protein:
Fat:
Vegetables:
Dairy:
Fiber:

Grains:

How many water intake:

◯ ◯ ◯ ◯ ◯ ◯ ◯ ◯

How hungry were you before eating?

How full were you after eating?

Notes

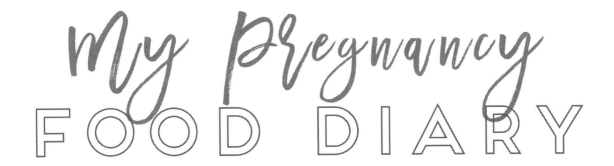

My Pregnancy
FOOD DIARY

Date: _____

Breakfast

Name:

Serving:

Calories:

Carbohydrates:

Protein:

Fat:

Vegetables:

Dairy:

Fiber:

Grains:

How many water intake:

◯ ◯ ◯ ◯ ◯ ◯ ◯ ◯

How hungry were you before eating?

How full were you after eating?

Lunch

Name:
Serving:
Calories:
Carbohydrates:
Protein:
Fat:
Vegetables:
Dairy:
Fiber:

Grains:

How many water intake:

◯　◯　◯　◯　◯　◯　◯　◯

How hungry were you before eating?

How full were you after eating?

Snacks

Name:
Serving:
Calories:
Carbohydrates:
Protein:
Fat:
Vegetables:
Dairy:
Fiber:

Grains:

How many water intake:

○ ○ ○ ○ ○ ○ ○ ○

How hungry were you before eating?

How full were you after eating?

Dinner

Name:
Serving:
Calories:
Carbohydrates:
Protein:
Fat:
Vegetables:
Dairy:
Fiber:

Grains:

How many water intake:

How hungry were you before eating?

How full were you after eating?

Notes

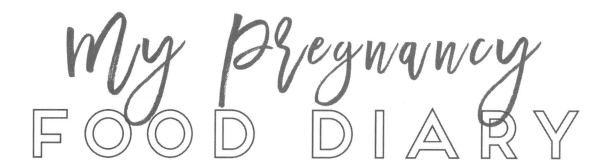

My Pregnancy
FOOD DIARY

Date: _____

Breakfast

Name:

Serving:

Calories:

Carbohydrates:

Protein:

Fat:

Vegetables:

Dairy:

Fiber:

Grains:

How many water intake:

◯ ◯ ◯ ◯ ◯ ◯ ◯ ◯

How hungry were you before eating?

How full were you after eating?

Lunch

Name:

Serving:

Calories:

Carbohydrates:

Protein:

Fat:

Vegetables:

Dairy:

Fiber:

Grains:

How many water intake:

◯ ◯ ◯ ◯ ◯ ◯ ◯ ◯

How hungry were you before eating?

How full were you after eating?

Snacks

Name:
Serving:
Calories:
Carbohydrates:
Protein:
Fat:
Vegetables:
Dairy:
Fiber:

Grains:

How many water intake:

○ ○ ○ ○ ○ ○ ○ ○

How hungry were you before eating?

How full were you after eating?

Dinner

Name:
Serving:
Calories:
Carbohydrates:
Protein:
Fat:
Vegetables:
Dairy:
Fiber:

Grains:

How many water intake:

◯ ◯ ◯ ◯ ◯ ◯ ◯ ◯

How hungry were you before eating?

How full were you after eating?

Notes

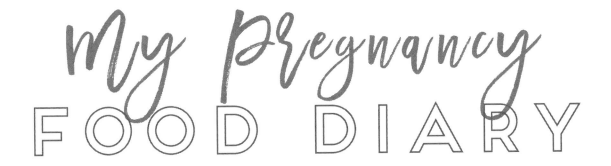

My Pregnancy
FOOD DIARY

Date: _____

Breakfast

Name:

Serving:

Calories:

Carbohydrates:

Protein:

Fat:

Vegetables:

Dairy:

Fiber:

Grains:

How many water intake:

◯ ◯ ◯ ◯ ◯ ◯ ◯ ◯

How hungry were you before eating?

How full were you after eating?

Lunch

Name:

Serving:

Calories:

Carbohydrates:

Protein:

Fat:

Vegetables:

Dairy:

Fiber:

Grains:

How many water intake:

◯ ◯ ◯ ◯ ◯ ◯ ◯ ◯

How hungry were you before eating?

How full were you after eating?

Snacks

Name:
Serving:
Calories:
Carbohydrates:
Protein:
Fat:
Vegetables:
Dairy:
Fiber:

Grains:

How many water intake:

○ ○ ○ ○ ○ ○ ○ ○

How hungry were you before eating?

How full were you after eating?

Dinner

Name:
Serving:
Calories:
Carbohydrates:
Protein:
Fat:
Vegetables:
Dairy:
Fiber:

Grains:

How many water intake:

◯ ◯ ◯ ◯ ◯ ◯ ◯ ◯

How hungry were you before eating?

How full were you after eating?

Notes

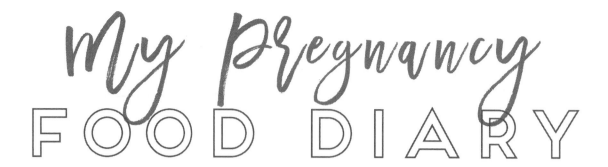

My Pregnancy
FOOD DIARY

Date: _____

Breakfast

Name:

Serving:

Calories:

Carbohydrates:

Protein:

Fat:

Vegetables:

Dairy:

Fiber:

Grains:

How many water intake:

◯ ◯ ◯ ◯ ◯ ◯ ◯ ◯

How hungry were you before eating?

How full were you after eating?

Lunch

Name:
Serving:
Calories:
Carbohydrates:
Protein:
Fat:
Vegetables:
Dairy:
Fiber:

Grains:

How many water intake:

○ ○ ○ ○ ○ ○ ○ ○

How hungry were you before eating?

How full were you after eating?

Snacks

Name:
Serving:
Calories:
Carbohydrates:
Protein:
Fat:
Vegetables:
Dairy:
Fiber:

Grains:

How many water intake:

◯ ◯ ◯ ◯ ◯ ◯ ◯ ◯

How hungry were you before eating?

How full were you after eating?

Dinner

Name:
Serving:
Calories:
Carbohydrates:
Protein:
Fat:
Vegetables:
Dairy:
Fiber:

Grains:

How many water intake:

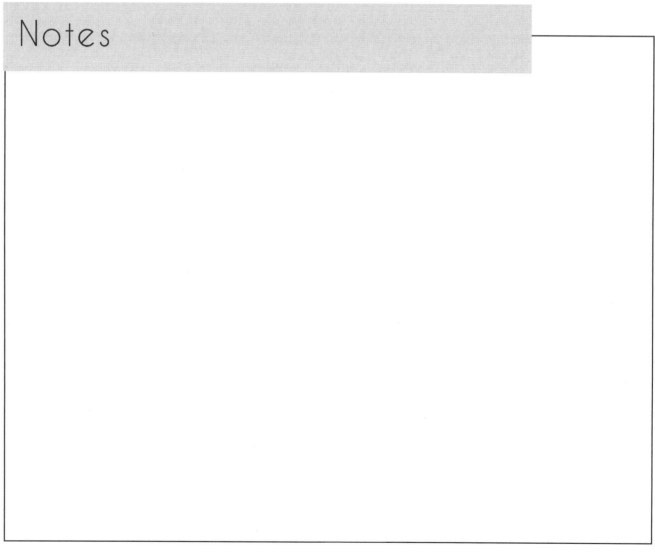

◯ ◯ ◯ ◯ ◯ ◯ ◯ ◯

How hungry were you before eating?

How full were you after eating?

Notes

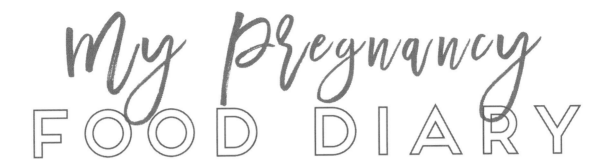

My Pregnancy
FOOD DIARY

Date: _____

Breakfast

Name:

Serving:

Calories:

Carbohydrates:

Protein:

Fat:

Vegetables:

Dairy:

Fiber:

Grains:

How many water intake:

○ ○ ○ ○ ○ ○ ○ ○

How hungry were you before eating?

How full were you after eating?

Lunch

Name:
Serving:
Calories:
Carbohydrates:
Protein:
Fat:
Vegetables:
Dairy:
Fiber:

Grains:

How many water intake:

◯　◯　◯　◯　◯　◯　◯　◯

How hungry were you before eating?

How full were you after eating?

Snacks

Name:

Serving:

Calories:

Carbohydrates:

Protein:

Fat:

Vegetables:

Dairy:

Fiber:

Grains:

How many water intake:

◯ ◯ ◯ ◯ ◯ ◯ ◯ ◯

How hungry were you before eating?

How full were you after eating?

Dinner

Name:

Serving:

Calories:

Carbohydrates:

Protein:

Fat:

Vegetables:

Dairy:

Fiber:

Grains:

How many water intake:

○ ○ ○ ○ ○ ○ ○ ○

How hungry were you before eating?

How full were you after eating?

Notes

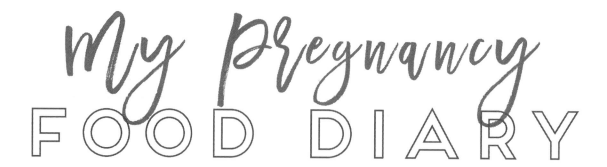

My Pregnancy
FOOD DIARY

Date: _____

Breakfast

Name:

Serving:

Calories:

Carbohydrates:

Protein:

Fat:

Vegetables:

Dairy:

Fiber:

Grains:

How many water intake:

◯ ◯ ◯ ◯ ◯ ◯ ◯ ◯

How hungry were you before eating?

How full were you after eating?

Lunch

Name:

Serving:

Calories:

Carbohydrates:

Protein:

Fat:

Vegetables:

Dairy:

Fiber:

Grains:

How many water intake:

◯ ◯ ◯ ◯ ◯ ◯ ◯ ◯

How hungry were you before eating?

How full were you after eating?

Snacks

Name:

Serving:

Calories:

Carbohydrates:

Protein:

Fat:

Vegetables:

Dairy:

Fiber:

Grains:

How many water intake:

◯ ◯ ◯ ◯ ◯ ◯ ◯ ◯

How hungry were you before eating?

How full were you after eating?

Dinner

Name:
Serving:
Calories:
Carbohydrates:
Protein:
Fat:
Vegetables:
Dairy:
Fiber:

Grains:

How many water intake:

◯ ◯ ◯ ◯ ◯ ◯ ◯ ◯

How hungry were you before eating?

How full were you after eating?

Notes

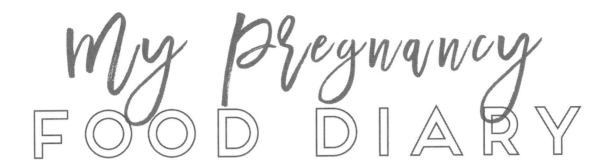

My Pregnancy
FOOD DIARY

Date: _____

Breakfast

Name:

Serving:

Calories:

Carbohydrates:

Protein:

Fat:

Vegetables:

Dairy:

Fiber:

Grains:

How many water intake:

◯ ◯ ◯ ◯ ◯ ◯ ◯ ◯

How hungry were you before eating?

How full were you after eating?

Lunch

Name:

Serving:

Calories:

Carbohydrates:

Protein:

Fat:

Vegetables:

Dairy:

Fiber:

Grains:

How many water intake:

◯ ◯ ◯ ◯ ◯ ◯ ◯ ◯

How hungry were you before eating?

How full were you after eating?

Snacks

Name:
Serving:
Calories:
Carbohydrates:
Protein:
Fat:
Vegetables:
Dairy:
Fiber:

Grains:

How many water intake:

$\bigcirc \quad \bigcirc \quad \bigcirc \quad \bigcirc \quad \bigcirc \quad \bigcirc \quad \bigcirc \quad \bigcirc$

How hungry were you before eating?

How full were you after eating?

Dinner

Name:

Serving:

Calories:

Carbohydrates:

Protein:

Fat:

Vegetables:

Dairy:

Fiber:

Grains:

How many water intake:

◯ ◯ ◯ ◯ ◯ ◯ ◯ ◯

How hungry were you before eating?

How full were you after eating?

Notes

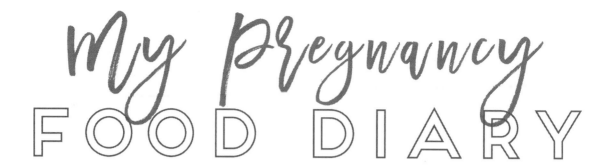

My Pregnancy
FOOD DIARY

Date: _____

Breakfast

Name:

Serving:

Calories:

Carbohydrates:

Protein:

Fat:

Vegetables:

Dairy:

Fiber:

Grains:

How many water intake:

◯ ◯ ◯ ◯ ◯ ◯ ◯ ◯

How hungry were you before eating?

How full were you after eating?

Lunch

Name:
Serving:
Calories:
Carbohydrates:
Protein:
Fat:
Vegetables:
Dairy:
Fiber:

Grains:

How many water intake:

◯ ◯ ◯ ◯ ◯ ◯ ◯ ◯

How hungry were you before eating?

How full were you after eating?

Snacks

Name:

Serving:

Calories:

Carbohydrates:

Protein:

Fat:

Vegetables:

Dairy:

Fiber:

Grains:

How many water intake:

◯ ◯ ◯ ◯ ◯ ◯ ◯ ◯

How hungry were you before eating?

How full were you after eating?

Dinner

Name:
Serving:
Calories:
Carbohydrates:
Protein:
Fat:
Vegetables:
Dairy:
Fiber:

Grains:

How many water intake:

◯ ◯ ◯ ◯ ◯ ◯ ◯ ◯

How hungry were you before eating?

How full were you after eating?

Notes

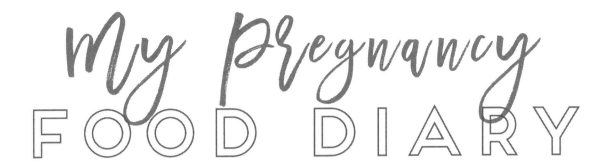

My Pregnancy
FOOD DIARY

Date: _____

Breakfast

Name:

Serving:

Calories:

Carbohydrates:

Protein:

Fat:

Vegetables:

Dairy:

Fiber:

Grains:

How many water intake:

◯ ◯ ◯ ◯ ◯ ◯ ◯ ◯

How hungry were you before eating?

How full were you after eating?

Lunch

Name:

Serving:

Calories:

Carbohydrates:

Protein:

Fat:

Vegetables:

Dairy:

Fiber:

Grains:

How many water intake:

○ ○ ○ ○ ○ ○ ○ ○

How hungry were you before eating?

How full were you after eating?

Snacks

Name:
Serving:
Calories:
Carbohydrates:
Protein:
Fat:
Vegetables:
Dairy:
Fiber:

Grains:

How many water intake:

◯ ◯ ◯ ◯ ◯ ◯ ◯ ◯

How hungry were you before eating?

How full were you after eating?

Dinner

Name:
Serving:
Calories:
Carbohydrates:
Protein:
Fat:
Vegetables:
Dairy:
Fiber:

Grains:

How many water intake:

◯ ◯ ◯ ◯ ◯ ◯ ◯ ◯

How hungry were you before eating?

How full were you after eating?

Notes

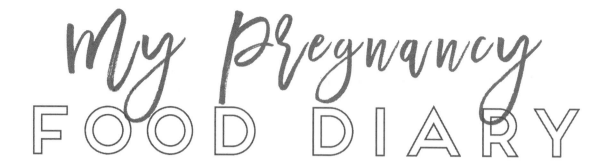

My Pregnancy
FOOD DIARY

Date: _____

Breakfast

Name:

Serving:

Calories:

Carbohydrates:

Protein:

Fat:

Vegetables:

Dairy:

Fiber:

Grains:

How many water intake:

○ ○ ○ ○ ○ ○ ○ ○

How hungry were you before eating?

How full were you after eating?

Lunch

Name:
Serving:
Calories:
Carbohydrates:
Protein:
Fat:
Vegetables:
Dairy:
Fiber:

Grains:

How many water intake:

◯ ◯ ◯ ◯ ◯ ◯ ◯ ◯

How hungry were you before eating?

How full were you after eating?

Snacks

Name:
Serving:
Calories:
Carbohydrates:
Protein:
Fat:
Vegetables:
Dairy:
Fiber:

Grains:

How many water intake:

◯ ◯ ◯ ◯ ◯ ◯ ◯ ◯

How hungry were you before eating?

How full were you after eating?

Dinner

Name:

Serving:

Calories:

Carbohydrates:

Protein:

Fat:

Vegetables:

Dairy:

Fiber:

Grains:

How many water intake:

○ ○ ○ ○ ○ ○ ○ ○

How hungry were you before eating?

How full were you after eating?

Notes

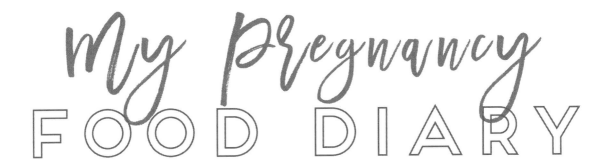

My Pregnancy
FOOD DIARY

Date: _____

Breakfast

Name:

Serving:

Calories:

Carbohydrates:

Protein:

Fat:

Vegetables:

Dairy:

Fiber:

Grains:

How many water intake:

◯ ◯ ◯ ◯ ◯ ◯ ◯ ◯

How hungry were you before eating?

How full were you after eating?

Lunch

Name:
Serving:
Calories:
Carbohydrates:
Protein:
Fat:
Vegetables:
Dairy:
Fiber:

Grains:

How many water intake:

◯ ◯ ◯ ◯ ◯ ◯ ◯ ◯

How hungry were you before eating?

How full were you after eating?

Snacks

Name:
Serving:
Calories:
Carbohydrates:
Protein:
Fat:
Vegetables:
Dairy:
Fiber:

Grains:

How many water intake:

◯ ◯ ◯ ◯ ◯ ◯ ◯ ◯

How hungry were you before eating?

How full were you after eating?

Dinner

Name:
Serving:
Calories:
Carbohydrates:
Protein:
Fat:
Vegetables:
Dairy:
Fiber:

Grains:

How many water intake:

How hungry were you before eating?

How full were you after eating?

Notes

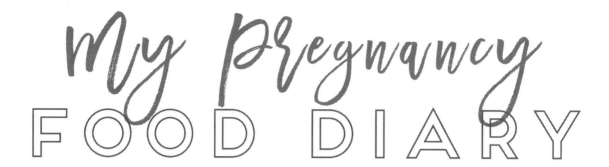

My Pregnancy
FOOD DIARY

Date: _____

Breakfast

Name:

Serving:

Calories:

Carbohydrates:

Protein:

Fat:

Vegetables:

Dairy:

Fiber:

Grains:

How many water intake:

◯ ◯ ◯ ◯ ◯ ◯ ◯ ◯

How hungry were you before eating?

How full were you after eating?

Lunch

Name:
Serving:
Calories:
Carbohydrates:
Protein:
Fat:
Vegetables:
Dairy:
Fiber:

Grains:

How many water intake:

◯ ◯ ◯ ◯ ◯ ◯ ◯ ◯

How hungry were you before eating?

How full were you after eating?

Snacks

Name:
Serving:
Calories:
Carbohydrates:
Protein:
Fat:
Vegetables:
Dairy:
Fiber:

Grains:

How many water intake:

◯ ◯ ◯ ◯ ◯ ◯ ◯ ◯

How hungry were you before eating?

How full were you after eating?

Dinner

Name:
Serving:
Calories:
Carbohydrates:
Protein:
Fat:
Vegetables:
Dairy:
Fiber:

Grains:

How many water intake:

◯ ◯ ◯ ◯ ◯ ◯ ◯ ◯

How hungry were you before eating?

How full were you after eating?

Notes

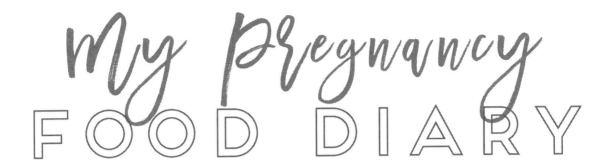

My Pregnancy
FOOD DIARY

Date: _____

Breakfast

Name:

Serving:

Calories:

Carbohydrates:

Protein:

Fat:

Vegetables:

Dairy:

Fiber:

Grains:

How many water intake:

○ ○ ○ ○ ○ ○ ○ ○

How hungry were you before eating?

How full were you after eating?

Lunch

Name:
Serving:
Calories:
Carbohydrates:
Protein:
Fat:
Vegetables:
Dairy:
Fiber:

Grains:

How many water intake:

○ ○ ○ ○ ○ ○ ○ ○

How hungry were you before eating?

How full were you after eating?

Snacks

Name:
Serving:
Calories:
Carbohydrates:
Protein:
Fat:
Vegetables:
Dairy:
Fiber:

Grains:

How many water intake:

○ ○ ○ ○ ○ ○ ○ ○

How hungry were you before eating?

How full were you after eating?

Dinner

Name:

Serving:

Calories:

Carbohydrates:

Protein:

Fat:

Vegetables:

Dairy:

Fiber:

Grains:

How many water intake:

○ ○ ○ ○ ○ ○ ○ ○

How hungry were you before eating?

How full were you after eating?

Notes

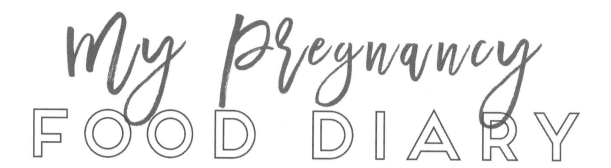

My Pregnancy
FOOD DIARY

Date: _____

Breakfast

Name:

Serving:

Calories:

Carbohydrates:

Protein:

Fat:

Vegetables:

Dairy:

Fiber:

Grains:

How many water intake:

○ ○ ○ ○ ○ ○ ○ ○

How hungry were you before eating?

How full were you after eating?

Lunch

Name:
Serving:
Calories:
Carbohydrates:
Protein:
Fat:
Vegetables:
Dairy:
Fiber:

Grains:

How many water intake:

◯ ◯ ◯ ◯ ◯ ◯ ◯ ◯

How hungry were you before eating?

How full were you after eating?

Snacks

Name:
Serving:
Calories:
Carbohydrates:
Protein:
Fat:
Vegetables:
Dairy:
Fiber:

Grains:

How many water intake:

◯ ◯ ◯ ◯ ◯ ◯ ◯ ◯

How hungry were you before eating?

How full were you after eating?

Dinner

Name:
Serving:
Calories:
Carbohydrates:
Protein:
Fat:
Vegetables:
Dairy:
Fiber:

Grains:

How many water intake:

◯ ◯ ◯ ◯ ◯ ◯ ◯ ◯

How hungry were you before eating?

How full were you after eating?

Notes

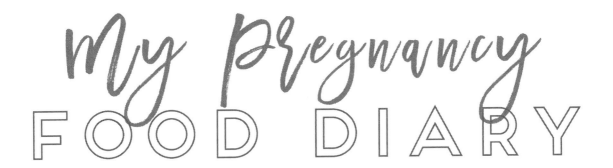

My Pregnancy
FOOD DIARY

Date: _____

Breakfast

Name:

Serving:

Calories:

Carbohydrates:

Protein:

Fat:

Vegetables:

Dairy:

Fiber:

Grains:

How many water intake:

◯ ◯ ◯ ◯ ◯ ◯ ◯ ◯

How hungry were you before eating?

How full were you after eating?

Lunch

Name:

Serving:

Calories:

Carbohydrates:

Protein:

Fat:

Vegetables:

Dairy:

Fiber:

Grains:

How many water intake:

◯ ◯ ◯ ◯ ◯ ◯ ◯ ◯

How hungry were you before eating?

How full were you after eating?

Snacks

Name:
Serving:
Calories:
Carbohydrates:
Protein:
Fat:
Vegetables:
Dairy:
Fiber:

Grains:

How many water intake:

○ ○ ○ ○ ○ ○ ○ ○

How hungry were you before eating?

How full were you after eating?

Dinner

Name:

Serving:

Calories:

Carbohydrates:

Protein:

Fat:

Vegetables:

Dairy:

Fiber:

Grains:

How many water intake:

◯ ◯ ◯ ◯ ◯ ◯ ◯ ◯

How hungry were you before eating?

How full were you after eating?

Notes

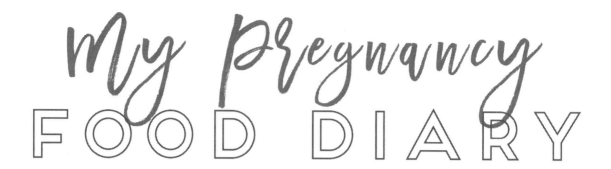

My Pregnancy
FOOD DIARY

Date: _____

Breakfast

Name:

Serving:

Calories:

Carbohydrates:

Protein:

Fat:

Vegetables:

Dairy:

Fiber:

Grains:

How many water intake:

◯ ◯ ◯ ◯ ◯ ◯ ◯ ◯

How hungry were you before eating?

How full were you after eating?

Lunch

Name:
Serving:
Calories:
Carbohydrates:
Protein:
Fat:
Vegetables:
Dairy:
Fiber:

Grains:

How many water intake:

◯ ◯ ◯ ◯ ◯ ◯ ◯ ◯

How hungry were you before eating?

How full were you after eating?

Snacks

Name:
Serving:
Calories:
Carbohydrates:
Protein:
Fat:
Vegetables:
Dairy:
Fiber:

Grains:

How many water intake:

○ ○ ○ ○ ○ ○ ○ ○

How hungry were you before eating?

How full were you after eating?

Dinner

Name:
Serving:
Calories:
Carbohydrates:
Protein:
Fat:
Vegetables:
Dairy:
Fiber:

Grains:

How many water intake:

◯ ◯ ◯ ◯ ◯ ◯ ◯ ◯

How hungry were you before eating?

How full were you after eating?

Notes

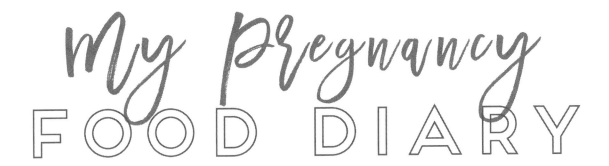

My Pregnancy
FOOD DIARY

Date: _____

Breakfast

Name:

Serving:

Calories:

Carbohydrates:

Protein:

Fat:

Vegetables:

Dairy:

Fiber:

Grains:

How many water intake:

○ ○ ○ ○ ○ ○ ○ ○

How hungry were you before eating?

How full were you after eating?

Lunch

Name:

Serving:

Calories:

Carbohydrates:

Protein:

Fat:

Vegetables:

Dairy:

Fiber:

Grains:

How many water intake:

○　○　○　○　○　○　○　○

How hungry were you before eating?

How full were you after eating?

Snacks

Name:
Serving:
Calories:
Carbohydrates:
Protein:
Fat:
Vegetables:
Dairy:
Fiber:

Grains:

How many water intake:

◯ ◯ ◯ ◯ ◯ ◯ ◯ ◯

How hungry were you before eating?

How full were you after eating?

Dinner

Name:
Serving:
Calories:
Carbohydrates:
Protein:
Fat:
Vegetables:
Dairy:
Fiber:

Grains:

How many water intake:

◯ ◯ ◯ ◯ ◯ ◯ ◯ ◯

How hungry were you before eating?

How full were you after eating?

Notes

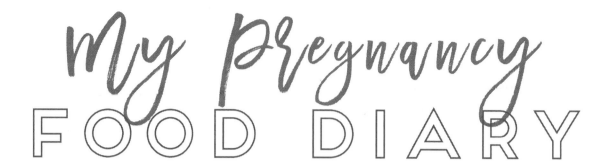

My Pregnancy
FOOD DIARY

Date: _____

Breakfast

Name:

Serving:

Calories:

Carbohydrates:

Protein:

Fat:

Vegetables:

Dairy:

Fiber:

Grains:

How many water intake:

○ ○ ○ ○ ○ ○ ○ ○

How hungry were you before eating?

How full were you after eating?

Lunch

Name:

Serving:

Calories:

Carbohydrates:

Protein:

Fat:

Vegetables:

Dairy:

Fiber:

Grains:

How many water intake:

○ ○ ○ ○ ○ ○ ○ ○

How hungry were you before eating?

How full were you after eating?

Snacks

Name:
Serving:
Calories:
Carbohydrates:
Protein:
Fat:
Vegetables:
Dairy:
Fiber:

Grains:

How many water intake:

◯ ◯ ◯ ◯ ◯ ◯ ◯ ◯

How hungry were you before eating?

How full were you after eating?

Dinner

Name:

Serving:

Calories:

Carbohydrates:

Protein:

Fat:

Vegetables:

Dairy:

Fiber:

Grains:

How many water intake:

◯ ◯ ◯ ◯ ◯ ◯ ◯ ◯

How hungry were you before eating?

How full were you after eating?

Notes

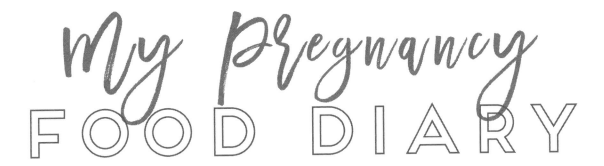

My Pregnancy
FOOD DIARY

Date: _____

Breakfast

Name:

Serving:

Calories:

Carbohydrates:

Protein:

Fat:

Vegetables:

Dairy:

Fiber:

Grains:

How many water intake:

◯ ◯ ◯ ◯ ◯ ◯ ◯ ◯

How hungry were you before eating?

How full were you after eating?

Lunch

Name:

Serving:

Calories:

Carbohydrates:

Protein:

Fat:

Vegetables:

Dairy:

Fiber:

Grains:

How many water intake:

○ ○ ○ ○ ○ ○ ○ ○

How hungry were you before eating?

How full were you after eating?

Snacks

Name:
Serving:
Calories:
Carbohydrates:
Protein:
Fat:
Vegetables:
Dairy:
Fiber:

Grains:

How many water intake:

◯ ◯ ◯ ◯ ◯ ◯ ◯ ◯

How hungry were you before eating?

How full were you after eating?

Dinner

Name:
Serving:
Calories:
Carbohydrates:
Protein:
Fat:
Vegetables:
Dairy:
Fiber:

Grains:

How many water intake:

◯ ◯ ◯ ◯ ◯ ◯ ◯ ◯

How hungry were you before eating?

How full were you after eating?

Notes

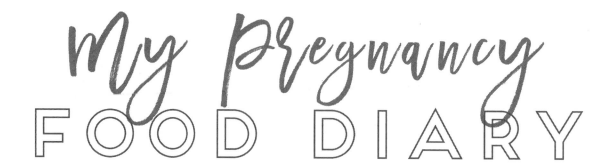

My Pregnancy FOOD DIARY

Date: _____

Breakfast

Name:

Serving:

Calories:

Carbohydrates:

Protein:

Fat:

Vegetables:

Dairy:

Fiber:

Grains:

How many water intake:

◯ ◯ ◯ ◯ ◯ ◯ ◯ ◯

How hungry were you before eating?

How full were you after eating?

Lunch

Name:

Serving:

Calories:

Carbohydrates:

Protein:

Fat:

Vegetables:

Dairy:

Fiber:

Grains:

How many water intake:

◯ ◯ ◯ ◯ ◯ ◯ ◯ ◯

How hungry were you before eating?

How full were you after eating?

Snacks

Name:
Serving:
Calories:
Carbohydrates:
Protein:
Fat:
Vegetables:
Dairy:
Fiber:

Grains:

How many water intake:

◯ ◯ ◯ ◯ ◯ ◯ ◯ ◯

How hungry were you before eating?

How full were you after eating?

Dinner

Name:
Serving:
Calories:
Carbohydrates:
Protein:
Fat:
Vegetables:
Dairy:
Fiber:

Grains:

How many water intake:

◯ ◯ ◯ ◯ ◯ ◯ ◯ ◯

How hungry were you before eating?

How full were you after eating?

Notes

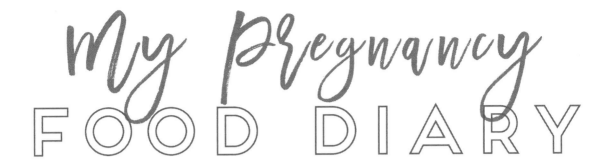

My Pregnancy
FOOD DIARY

Date: _____

Breakfast

Name:

Serving:

Calories:

Carbohydrates:

Protein:

Fat:

Vegetables:

Dairy:

Fiber:

Grains:

How many water intake:

◯ ◯ ◯ ◯ ◯ ◯ ◯ ◯

How hungry were you before eating?

How full were you after eating?

Lunch

Name:

Serving:

Calories:

Carbohydrates:

Protein:

Fat:

Vegetables:

Dairy:

Fiber:

Grains:

How many water intake:

◯ ◯ ◯ ◯ ◯ ◯ ◯ ◯

How hungry were you before eating?

How full were you after eating?

Snacks

Name:
Serving:
Calories:
Carbohydrates:
Protein:
Fat:
Vegetables:
Dairy:
Fiber:

Grains:

How many water intake:

◯ ◯ ◯ ◯ ◯ ◯ ◯ ◯

How hungry were you before eating?

How full were you after eating?

Dinner

Name:
Serving:
Calories:
Carbohydrates:
Protein:
Fat:
Vegetables:
Dairy:
Fiber:

Grains:

How many water intake:

How hungry were you before eating?

How full were you after eating?

Notes

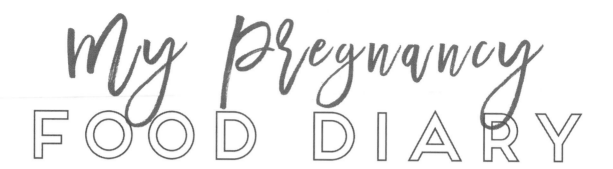

My Pregnancy
FOOD DIARY

Date: _____

Breakfast

Name:

Serving:

Calories:

Carbohydrates:

Protein:

Fat:

Vegetables:

Dairy:

Fiber:

Grains:

How many water intake:

◯ ◯ ◯ ◯ ◯ ◯ ◯ ◯

How hungry were you before eating?

How full were you after eating?

Lunch

Name:
Serving:
Calories:
Carbohydrates:
Protein:
Fat:
Vegetables:
Dairy:
Fiber:

Grains:

How many water intake:

◯ ◯ ◯ ◯ ◯ ◯ ◯ ◯

How hungry were you before eating?

How full were you after eating?

Snacks

Name:
Serving:
Calories:
Carbohydrates:
Protein:
Fat:
Vegetables:
Dairy:
Fiber:

Grains:

How many water intake:

◯ ◯ ◯ ◯ ◯ ◯ ◯ ◯

How hungry were you before eating?

How full were you after eating?

Dinner

Name:

Serving:

Calories:

Carbohydrates:

Protein:

Fat:

Vegetables:

Dairy:

Fiber:

Grains:

How many water intake:

◯ ◯ ◯ ◯ ◯ ◯ ◯ ◯

How hungry were you before eating?

How full were you after eating?

Notes

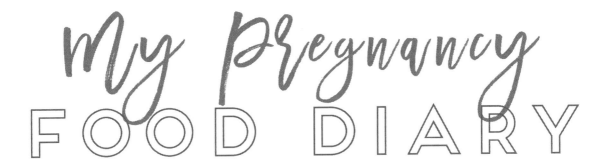

My Pregnancy
FOOD DIARY

Date: _____

Breakfast

Name:

Serving:

Calories:

Carbohydrates:

Protein:

Fat:

Vegetables:

Dairy:

Fiber:

Grains:

How many water intake:

○ ○ ○ ○ ○ ○ ○ ○

How hungry were you before eating?

How full were you after eating?

Lunch

Name:
Serving:
Calories:
Carbohydrates:
Protein:
Fat:
Vegetables:
Dairy:
Fiber:

Grains:

How many water intake:

◯ ◯ ◯ ◯ ◯ ◯ ◯ ◯

How hungry were you before eating?

How full were you after eating?

Snacks

Name:
Serving:
Calories:
Carbohydrates:
Protein:
Fat:
Vegetables:
Dairy:
Fiber:

Grains:

How many water intake:

◯ ◯ ◯ ◯ ◯ ◯ ◯ ◯

How hungry were you before eating?

How full were you after eating?

Dinner

Name:
Serving:
Calories:
Carbohydrates:
Protein:
Fat:
Vegetables:
Dairy:
Fiber:

Grains:

How many water intake:

◯ ◯ ◯ ◯ ◯ ◯ ◯ ◯

How hungry were you before eating?

How full were you after eating?

Notes

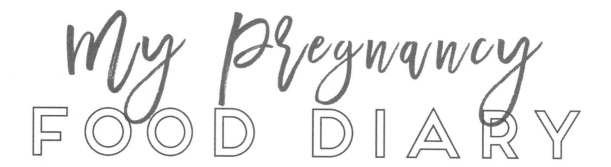

My Pregnancy
FOOD DIARY

Date: _____

Breakfast

Name:

Serving:

Calories:

Carbohydrates:

Protein:

Fat:

Vegetables:

Dairy:

Fiber:

Grains:

How many water intake:

◯ ◯ ◯ ◯ ◯ ◯ ◯ ◯

How hungry were you before eating?

How full were you after eating?

Lunch

Name:
Serving:
Calories:
Carbohydrates:
Protein:
Fat:
Vegetables:
Dairy:
Fiber:

Grains:

How many water intake:

◯ ◯ ◯ ◯ ◯ ◯ ◯ ◯

How hungry were you before eating?

How full were you after eating?

Snacks

Name:
Serving:
Calories:
Carbohydrates:
Protein:
Fat:
Vegetables:
Dairy:
Fiber:

Grains:

How many water intake:

○ ○ ○ ○ ○ ○ ○ ○

How hungry were you before eating?

How full were you after eating?

Dinner

Name:

Serving:

Calories:

Carbohydrates:

Protein:

Fat:

Vegetables:

Dairy:

Fiber:

Grains:

How many water intake:

◯ ◯ ◯ ◯ ◯ ◯ ◯ ◯

How hungry were you before eating?

How full were you after eating?

Notes

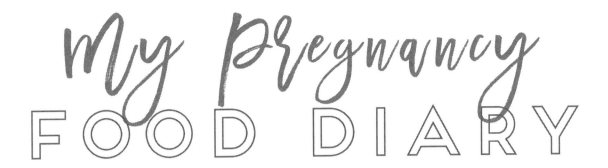

My Pregnancy
FOOD DIARY

Date: _____

Breakfast

Name:

Serving:

Calories:

Carbohydrates:

Protein:

Fat:

Vegetables:

Dairy:

Fiber:

Grains:

How many water intake:

◯ ◯ ◯ ◯ ◯ ◯ ◯ ◯

How hungry were you before eating?

How full were you after eating?

Lunch

Name:

Serving:

Calories:

Carbohydrates:

Protein:

Fat:

Vegetables:

Dairy:

Fiber:

Grains:

How many water intake:

○ ○ ○ ○ ○ ○ ○ ○

How hungry were you before eating?

How full were you after eating?

Snacks

Name:
Serving:
Calories:
Carbohydrates:
Protein:
Fat:
Vegetables:
Dairy:
Fiber:

Grains:

How many water intake:

◯ ◯ ◯ ◯ ◯ ◯ ◯ ◯

How hungry were you before eating?

How full were you after eating?

Dinner

Name:
Serving:
Calories:
Carbohydrates:
Protein:
Fat:
Vegetables:
Dairy:
Fiber:

Grains:

How many water intake:

◯ ◯ ◯ ◯ ◯ ◯ ◯ ◯

How hungry were you before eating?

How full were you after eating?

Notes

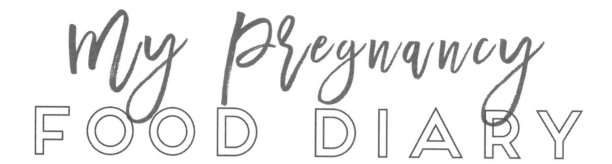
My Pregnancy
FOOD DIARY

Date: _____

Breakfast

Name:

Serving:

Calories:

Carbohydrates:

Protein:

Fat:

Vegetables:

Dairy:

Fiber:

Grains:

How many water intake:

◯ ◯ ◯ ◯ ◯ ◯ ◯ ◯

How hungry were you before eating?

How full were you after eating?

Lunch

Name:

Serving:

Calories:

Carbohydrates:

Protein:

Fat:

Vegetables:

Dairy:

Fiber:

Grains:

How many water intake:

○ ○ ○ ○ ○ ○ ○ ○

How hungry were you before eating?

How full were you after eating?

Snacks

Name:
Serving:
Calories:
Carbohydrates:
Protein:
Fat:
Vegetables:
Dairy:
Fiber:

Grains:

How many water intake:

○ ○ ○ ○ ○ ○ ○ ○

How hungry were you before eating?

How full were you after eating?

Dinner

Name:
Serving:
Calories:
Carbohydrates:
Protein:
Fat:
Vegetables:
Dairy:
Fiber:

Grains:

How many water intake:

◯ ◯ ◯ ◯ ◯ ◯ ◯ ◯

How hungry were you before eating?

How full were you after eating?

Notes

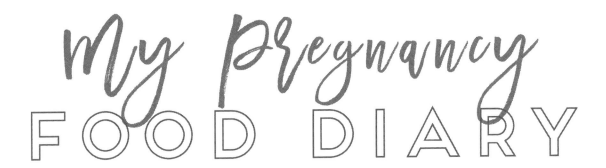

Date: _____

Breakfast

Name:

Serving:

Calories:

Carbohydrates:

Protein:

Fat:

Vegetables:

Dairy:

Fiber:

Grains:

How many water intake:

◯ ◯ ◯ ◯ ◯ ◯ ◯ ◯

How hungry were you before eating?

How full were you after eating?

Lunch

Name:
Serving:
Calories:
Carbohydrates:
Protein:
Fat:
Vegetables:
Dairy:
Fiber:

Grains:

How many water intake:

◯ ◯ ◯ ◯ ◯ ◯ ◯ ◯

How hungry were you before eating?

How full were you after eating?

Snacks

Name:
Serving:
Calories:
Carbohydrates:
Protein:
Fat:
Vegetables:
Dairy:
Fiber:

Grains:

How many water intake:

◯ ◯ ◯ ◯ ◯ ◯ ◯ ◯

How hungry were you before eating?

How full were you after eating?

Dinner

Name:
Serving:
Calories:
Carbohydrates:
Protein:
Fat:
Vegetables:
Dairy:
Fiber:

Grains:

How many water intake:

◯ ◯ ◯ ◯ ◯ ◯ ◯ ◯

How hungry were you before eating?

How full were you after eating?

Notes

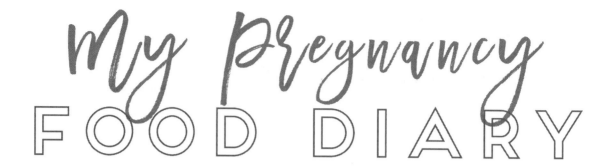

My Pregnancy
FOOD DIARY

Date: _____

Breakfast

Name:

Serving:

Calories:

Carbohydrates:

Protein:

Fat:

Vegetables:

Dairy:

Fiber:

Grains:

How many water intake:

◯ ◯ ◯ ◯ ◯ ◯ ◯ ◯

How hungry were you before eating?

How full were you after eating?

Lunch

Name:
Serving:
Calories:
Carbohydrates:
Protein:
Fat:
Vegetables:
Dairy:
Fiber:

Grains:

How many water intake:

◯ ◯ ◯ ◯ ◯ ◯ ◯ ◯

How hungry were you before eating?

How full were you after eating?

Snacks

Name:

Serving:

Calories:

Carbohydrates:

Protein:

Fat:

Vegetables:

Dairy:

Fiber:

Grains:

How many water intake:

◯ ◯ ◯ ◯ ◯ ◯ ◯ ◯

How hungry were you before eating?

How full were you after eating?

Dinner

Name:

Serving:

Calories:

Carbohydrates:

Protein:

Fat:

Vegetables:

Dairy:

Fiber:

Grains:

How many water intake:

◯ ◯ ◯ ◯ ◯ ◯ ◯ ◯

How hungry were you before eating?

How full were you after eating?

Notes

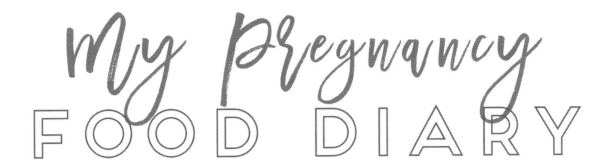

My Pregnancy
FOOD DIARY

Date: _____

Breakfast

Name:

Serving:

Calories:

Carbohydrates:

Protein:

Fat:

Vegetables:

Dairy:

Fiber:

Grains:

How many water intake:

◯ ◯ ◯ ◯ ◯ ◯ ◯ ◯

How hungry were you before eating?

How full were you after eating?

Lunch

Name:

Serving:

Calories:

Carbohydrates:

Protein:

Fat:

Vegetables:

Dairy:

Fiber:

Grains:

How many water intake:

◯ ◯ ◯ ◯ ◯ ◯ ◯ ◯

How hungry were you before eating?

How full were you after eating?

Snacks

Name:
Serving:
Calories:
Carbohydrates:
Protein:
Fat:
Vegetables:
Dairy:
Fiber:

Grains:

How many water intake:

○ ○ ○ ○ ○ ○ ○ ○

How hungry were you before eating?

How full were you after eating?

Dinner

Name:
Serving:
Calories:
Carbohydrates:
Protein:
Fat:
Vegetables:
Dairy:
Fiber:

Grains:

How many water intake:

○ ○ ○ ○ ○ ○ ○ ○

How hungry were you before eating?

How full were you after eating?

Notes

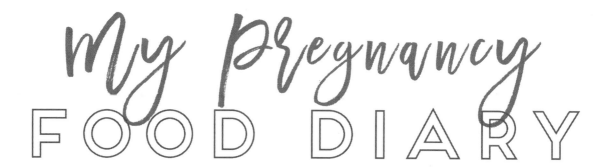

My Pregnancy
FOOD DIARY

Date: _____

Breakfast

Name:

Serving:

Calories:

Carbohydrates:

Protein:

Fat:

Vegetables:

Dairy:

Fiber:

Grains:

How many water intake:

◯ ◯ ◯ ◯ ◯ ◯ ◯ ◯

How hungry were you before eating?

How full were you after eating?

Lunch

Name:
Serving:
Calories:
Carbohydrates:
Protein:
Fat:
Vegetables:
Dairy:
Fiber:

Grains:

How many water intake:

○ ○ ○ ○ ○ ○ ○ ○

How hungry were you before eating?

How full were you after eating?

Snacks

Name:

Serving:

Calories:

Carbohydrates:

Protein:

Fat:

Vegetables:

Dairy:

Fiber:

Grains:

How many water intake:

◯ ◯ ◯ ◯ ◯ ◯ ◯ ◯

How hungry were you before eating?

How full were you after eating?

Dinner

Name:
Serving:
Calories:
Carbohydrates:
Protein:
Fat:
Vegetables:
Dairy:
Fiber:

Grains:

How many water intake:

◯ ◯ ◯ ◯ ◯ ◯ ◯ ◯

How hungry were you before eating?

How full were you after eating?

Notes

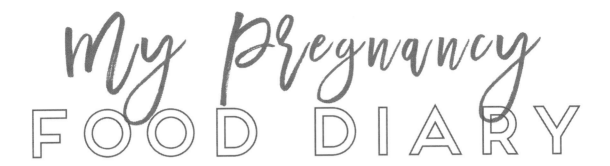

My Pregnancy
FOOD DIARY

Date: _____

Breakfast

Name:

Serving:

Calories:

Carbohydrates:

Protein:

Fat:

Vegetables:

Dairy:

Fiber:

Grains:

How many water intake:

◯ ◯ ◯ ◯ ◯ ◯ ◯ ◯

How hungry were you before eating?

How full were you after eating?

Lunch

Name:

Serving:

Calories:

Carbohydrates:

Protein:

Fat:

Vegetables:

Dairy:

Fiber:

Grains:

How many water intake:

◯ ◯ ◯ ◯ ◯ ◯ ◯ ◯

How hungry were you before eating?

How full were you after eating?

Snacks

Name:

Serving:

Calories:

Carbohydrates:

Protein:

Fat:

Vegetables:

Dairy:

Fiber:

Grains:

How many water intake:

○ ○ ○ ○ ○ ○ ○ ○

How hungry were you before eating?

How full were you after eating?

Dinner

Name:

Serving:

Calories:

Carbohydrates:

Protein:

Fat:

Vegetables:

Dairy:

Fiber:

Grains:

How many water intake:

◯ ◯ ◯ ◯ ◯ ◯ ◯ ◯

How hungry were you before eating?

How full were you after eating?

Notes

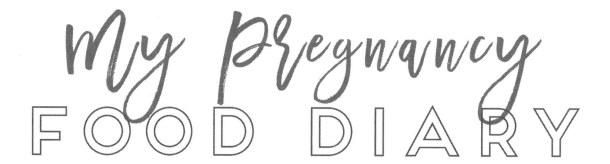

My Pregnancy
FOOD DIARY

Date: _____

Breakfast

Name:

Serving:

Calories:

Carbohydrates:

Protein:

Fat:

Vegetables:

Dairy:

Fiber:

Grains:

How many water intake:

◯ ◯ ◯ ◯ ◯ ◯ ◯ ◯

How hungry were you before eating?

How full were you after eating?

Lunch

Name:

Serving:

Calories:

Carbohydrates:

Protein:

Fat:

Vegetables:

Dairy:

Fiber:

Grains:

How many water intake:

◯ ◯ ◯ ◯ ◯ ◯ ◯ ◯

How hungry were you before eating?

How full were you after eating?

Snacks

Name:
Serving:
Calories:
Carbohydrates:
Protein:
Fat:
Vegetables:
Dairy:
Fiber:

Grains:

How many water intake:

○ ○ ○ ○ ○ ○ ○ ○

How hungry were you before eating?

How full were you after eating?

Dinner

Name:
Serving:
Calories:
Carbohydrates:
Protein:
Fat:
Vegetables:
Dairy:
Fiber:

Grains:

How many water intake:

○ ○ ○ ○ ○ ○ ○ ○

How hungry were you before eating?

How full were you after eating?

Notes

My Pregnancy
FOOD DIARY

Date: _____

Breakfast

Name:

Serving:

Calories:

Carbohydrates:

Protein:

Fat:

Vegetables:

Dairy:

Fiber:

Grains:

How many water intake:

◯ ◯ ◯ ◯ ◯ ◯ ◯ ◯

How hungry were you before eating?

How full were you after eating?

Lunch

Name:

Serving:

Calories:

Carbohydrates:

Protein:

Fat:

Vegetables:

Dairy:

Fiber:

Grains:

How many water intake:

◯ ◯ ◯ ◯ ◯ ◯ ◯ ◯

How hungry were you before eating?

How full were you after eating?

Snacks

Name:

Serving:

Calories:

Carbohydrates:

Protein:

Fat:

Vegetables:

Dairy:

Fiber:

Grains:

How many water intake:

○ ○ ○ ○ ○ ○ ○ ○

How hungry were you before eating?

How full were you after eating?

Dinner

Name:
Serving:
Calories:
Carbohydrates:
Protein:
Fat:
Vegetables:
Dairy:
Fiber:

Grains:

How many water intake:

◯ ◯ ◯ ◯ ◯ ◯ ◯ ◯

How hungry were you before eating?

How full were you after eating?

Notes

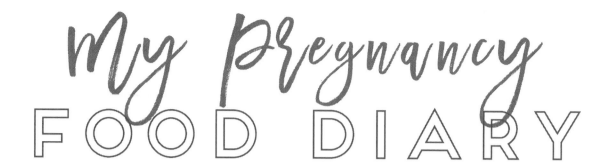

My Pregnancy
FOOD DIARY

Date: _____

Breakfast

Name:

Serving:

Calories:

Carbohydrates:

Protein:

Fat:

Vegetables:

Dairy:

Fiber:

Grains:

How many water intake:

◯ ◯ ◯ ◯ ◯ ◯ ◯ ◯

How hungry were you before eating?

How full were you after eating?

Lunch

Name:

Serving:

Calories:

Carbohydrates:

Protein:

Fat:

Vegetables:

Dairy:

Fiber:

Grains:

How many water intake:

◯ ◯ ◯ ◯ ◯ ◯ ◯ ◯

How hungry were you before eating?

How full were you after eating?

Snacks

Name:
Serving:
Calories:
Carbohydrates:
Protein:
Fat:
Vegetables:
Dairy:
Fiber:

Grains:

How many water intake:

◯ ◯ ◯ ◯ ◯ ◯ ◯ ◯

How hungry were you before eating?

How full were you after eating?

Dinner

Name:
Serving:
Calories:
Carbohydrates:
Protein:
Fat:
Vegetables:
Dairy:
Fiber:

Grains:

How many water intake:

◯ ◯ ◯ ◯ ◯ ◯ ◯ ◯

How hungry were you before eating?

How full were you after eating?

Notes

Made in the USA
Middletown, DE
30 June 2020

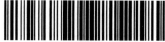

11576509R00179